FACING THE ENEMY:
Chronicles of a Cancer Doctor

Robert T. Wall Jr., M.D., F.A.C.P.

ISBN: 1503345556
ISBN 13: 9781503345553

For Susan, Spencer and Elizabeth

Table of Contents

Preface

This book is about the enemy, cancer, and how it affects real patients and their families. The book is written to help guide those who have just been diagnosed with cancer and those who want to know more about cancer; illustrates how cancer can be prevented and, if not prevented, how cancer can be treated. This book is about how the patient and family can survive the journey.

I also write this book for those already in medical training and for those who are considering entering the field of medicine. For them, I hope the stories illustrate that caring for the sick is the primary purpose of the practice of medicine. For these are not my stories but instead are the stories of patients and their families whose lives were changed forever by cancer. Their fears and anxieties are evident but so too is their courage and dignity in facing the enemy.

To effectively care for patients with cancer, the medical practitioner must keep current with a field that is rapidly changing because of advances in science and technology. The incredible changes in medicine I have seen over my forty year career provides testimony to that fact.

I am an oncologist and hematologist with long experience in diagnosing and treating cancer. I have been in academic medical centers and in private practice. I have seen firsthand the fear that the enemy causes; fear of learning that cancer is in the body, fear of treatment and fear for the future. Fear keeps some from seeking timely help. Fear leads others to demand unhelpful testing and treatment that diminishes their quality of life. To so many, cancer is the most dreaded unseen and unknowable enemy. In fact, a cancer diagnosis may not only lead to cure but may bring out the best and most noble acts in those facing the enemy. I hope the pages that follow will dispel the mystery about what cancer is, how cancer can be prevented and how cancer can be successfully treated.

My experience has taught me that an explanation of cancer and its treatment, using stories of others who have faced the same battle, is a useful way to help patients and their families. In this book, I have drawn on my experience in an attempt to explain the true nature of cancer and to demonstrate how advances in cancer prevention, diagnosis, and treatment have improved to the point that the enemy will soon be defeated.

I came to the study of oncology and hematology when these fields were just entering the modern era. The advancing science and the prospect of successfully helping patients with cancer was the attraction for me. The cancer could be seen under the microscope; the molecular derangements that caused the cancer could be dissected out; and, treatments were rapidly improving. I was also fortunate that the best teacher and clinician at my medical school was a hematologist who made the study fascinating and was able to vividly explain the field and offer a model of the physician I wanted to be: a skilled doctor who could provide a benefit to individuals and their families.

Today, the pace of change in the fields of oncology and hematology and indeed in all of medicine, from the scientific basis of practice to the ways in which health can be delivered to society, is accelerating. I hope that this book helps in understanding these changes.

The patient stories throughout this book reflect real situations and real outcomes. They are told as I recall them but of course without identification so that the people involved remain anonymous. I have been honored and humbled to have known these and all my patients and their families and I have been privileged to care for the hundreds who have sought my help in their most troubled time. I relate my journey as a doctor through the stories of my patients; each patient has changed me as a person and each has made me a better care giver. I hope these stories help others affected by cancer, help them face the fear and defeat the enemy.

one

Facing the Enemy

When I first met her, I was a new soldier in the cancer wars. This young woman, however, was a veteran; she had been facing the enemy for years. Now, she was in a hospital bed in a sterile ward dying from acute leukemia that had exploded out of her long standing chronic leukemia. I was a first year fellow in hematology and oncology and had just been assigned to her care. She and her family had been told by the attending physician that there was no further useful therapy. Although she had traveled from Wisconsin for experimental bone marrow therapy at our medical center, the treatment had not been successful and the decision was made that no further attempts at active cancer treatment would be given. The focus of her care was management of pain and anxiety. This was her status when I was assigned to her care as a first day, first year fellow.

This brave young patient radiated warmth and a joy of living despite all she had endured. She kept a sense of humor and had a tenacious attachment to each day remaining to her. We talked together about many things, including what we discovered was our favorite football team, the Green Bay Packers, and her favorite player, Bart Starr, who had been the team's quarterback some years before. I told her that I had become a Packers fan when, as a young boy, the head coach, who was a friend of my father's, invited me to sit on the team sidelines during a game played on the East Coast. After the game, the coach asked me what I thought of his team. The Packers had lost the game and the team was not yet the all-powerful team they were to become. I told the coach that his rookie quarterback, who had started the second half, had great promise. The young quarterback's name was Bart Starr and the coach was not nearly as sure as I was about his prospects. (Years later I met Bart Starr and told him the story of how I saved his career.) The patient was from Green Bay and was an avid fan. She and I laughed together at my personal contribution to the Green Bay Packers' success. Our shared stories and laughter gave her some comfort and happiness, triggering pleasant memories of a happier time far away from her hospital bed in an isolation unit.

The day came when I walked into her room as she was dying. She asked me to sit with her and hold her hand. She described what she was feeling as her final moments came. Within a short time, she told me that she could no longer see but she was not in pain. Then, she died. The experience of those last moments with this patient are never far from my mind. The sense of helplessness in the face of death, knowing that there is nothing more that can be done to treat the disease is a crushing weight on any doctor, perhaps especially on a young trainee. The patient and her family, however, saw it differently. They were thankful for the efforts to help her and the success in preventing any discomfort at the end.

This experience demonstrated that the patient is not defined by the disease. I had first decided to specialize in hematology and oncology because I was fascinated by the beauty and complexity of the blood system, and by the scientific and medical skills of a hematologist mentor in medical school. Viewing a blood sample spread on a glass slide and stained with colorful dyes to bring out the details of the blood cells appeared to me to reveal the secret of nature. Using the stained smear to diagnose a disorder was a powerful experience. In this instance, I could see this young woman's leukemia cells on the slide when I looked at her blood smear under the microscope. It all seemed so pure and straightforward. I learned, however, that the blood smear was not the person who had the disorder.

This young woman had a rich life with unique experiences and expectations. She had a family and friends. She had a hope for the future. In those moments when she felt fear, she was also very brave. She could not know how much I learned from her and how deeply my experience in caring for her affected me. My journey from trainee to doctor had begun in earnest. I would never be a disinterested physician dazzled by the beauty of the biology of human life; instead, I would endeavor to become a doctor who would comfort always and heal when possible. I would continue to learn all that I could about the field of hematology and oncology to be that physician. Going forward, I would see the individual first and use the knowledge that I had acquired to help the person however I could. I resolved to learn how to show patients that my purpose was to help and that their problems would be my problems as well. I would be their physician as well as their advocate. The patient would not struggle alone in this battle against the enemy.

I have repeatedly met and done battle with the enemy not only through treating my cancer patients but also in dealing with cancer in my own family. My son, my father, a sister, my wife's mother and my brother-in-law have each survived cancer.

My father had prostate cancer late in life. It was of a high grade and, if untreated, could have caused his death. Since he otherwise was in good health, I encouraged him to be treated even though the treatment would be difficult and potentially dangerous. I was able to guide his movement through the specialist maze and helped coordinate his radiation and antitestosterone treatment. Although he ultimately stopped his hormonal treatment because it made him "not feel himself" as he put it, the treatment was successful and the cancer never again became a health issue for him.

My sister and mother-in-law both developed breast cancer. The cancers were found during screening mammography. Both were small and had low-risk biological features. Each was treated with limited surgery to remove the tumor followed by radiation therapy to the breast. For a number of years after, each was placed on anti-estrogen therapy to suppress estrogen activity. Both have also remained free of cancer.

My brother-in-law developed a malignant melanoma of his ear. He was successfully treated by surgical removal of the tumor followed by surgical reconstruction of the ear. The ear reconstruction looked very natural and was done by a plastic surgeon who was a friend and medical school classmate. No other treatment was needed and he too remains well.

I understand the depth of shock and fear that a cancer diagnosis brings to a parent. Our son had testicular cancer, one of the most common cancers of young males. My wife and daughter and I were visiting him one weekend while he was in his first year of law school. He took me aside and told me that he had a swelling on one of his testicles. I knew the diagnosis immediately, even before examining him. Although I had treated many young men for testicular cancer, I felt a great apprehension in dealing with the disease so personally. Telling my wife and daughter was one of the most difficult tasks of my life. But, as with so many families, after the initial devastation, we quickly rallied and pledged to be positive and strong in supporting each other through the events to come.

At the time of our son's cancer diagnosis, there was some uncertainty among oncologists as to how to prevent a recurrence. Our son underwent limited surgery without additional treatment and all appeared successful. Traditionally, however, additional surgery was often advised to remove the abdominal lymph nodes. This recommendation was based on the premise that it would remove any cancer that might have spread but was too small to be detected on imaging studies, as well as to better stage the cancer and if further cancer was found, to initiate a course of chemotherapy for this potentially fast-growing and fast-spreading cancer.

For our son, I recommended aggressive surveillance with lab testing and CT scanning without additional surgery or chemotherapy. This recommendation was based on new studies in the field which showed that this approach could avoid the risks of chemotherapy and additional surgery. Chemotherapy and possibly additional surgery could be reserved for those with a high risk of recurrence based on the biology of the initial tumor or for those who had already developed metastatic disease or developed recurrent disease later.

Our son was very courageous in dealing with his cancer and never lost his sense of humor and love of life. He approached the disease with care in considering treatment options and discussed with me and his treating oncologist the various approaches and what was reflected in the studies in the field.

This was a very difficult time in the life of our family but it also brought us together and allowed us to recognize and appreciate the courage of not only the patient but each member of the family. We dealt with our fears by talking openly about our anxieties and considered together the best way forward. We pledged to see this through as a family and support one another. In the end, the decision was made to monitor his status closely and initiate treatment at the first sign of recurrence. A decade has passed without any signs of recurrence of the cancer. As a parent, the worry will always be there, but thankfully this threat seems to have passed.

These personal experiences with cancer in my family have added to my understanding of what every person experiences when facing the enemy. I hope that these experiences have made me a better physician and a better person. I see more clearly the needs of patients and their families and also recognize that with good advice and appropriate treatment, the chances of a successful battle with the enemy is high. Physicians must put the patient first and not miss each opportunity to serve those in need.

two

Good Morning, Reverend

My early career consisted of faculty appointments in hematology and oncology at two leading academic medical centers. Once my wife and I had children, we decided to move back to the city where I grew up, so that our children would be around extended family. For this transition, it was necessary that I enter the private practice of hematology and oncology. In this capacity, I treated patients in my office, as well as in several hospitals in the city. Hospital rounds began in the early morning so that I could arrive back at my office in time to see the first scheduled patient. I often rounded at the hospital again in the evening.

I was on call nights and weekends, with some breaks when other physicians would cover for me. Weekend and holiday rounds in the hospital often took all day, because of the number of patients to see and care for. Urgent situations were common during the day, requiring emergency room visits and return visits to the hospital to see new patients or to deal with critical matters.

Phone calls from the nursing staff at the hospital, other doctors, or from patients or their families at home continued through the night. My side of the phone discussions could be heard by my wife, and, over the years, she became knowledgeable in the language of medicine.

It was after a particularly long and difficult night on call, followed by long rounding at two hospitals, when I finally arrived in the room of a patient who was in the hospital because of an infection brought on by his multiple myeloma. This disease is a cancer of the plasma cells, which are blood cells that are a part of the immune system that normally fights off infection but that is profoundly weakened when multiple myeloma develops.

The patient's wife greeted me with "Doc, you are going to have a long life." I was very surprised by this statement but she explained that since it was late in the morning, she assumed that I had slept in and she concluded that I took good care of myself and got plenty of rest since I was seeing them so late in the morning. The truth was otherwise but her conclusion was understandable because she had no idea of the time needed to care for others.

In contrast, there were occasions when being at the patient's bedside too early in the morning was not warmly received. This could happen if I had been at the hospital through the night and made hospital rounds in the early morning hours before going to my office. I had a patient who, in self defense, knitted for me a stethoscope cover to keep the metal warm and minimize the shock of the cold instrument against her skin early in the morning. It also sometimes happened that I had to awaken patients and the family member who had decided to stay with the patient overnight. More than once a sleepy patient or family member saw my dark suit and tie and greeted me with the words "Morning, Reverend." Despite the identity confusion, it is true that the skills of a minister are necessary for the complete physician in comforting patients and families.

Treating the patient effectively always involves interaction with the family or friends who are a meaningful part of the patient's life. This can be especially challenging when the patient is a childhood friend or colleague. Every year, I still see in my office a friend from childhood who asked me many years ago to treat him for a large, high-risk melanoma on his back. When he contacted me, the cancer had spread to nearby lymph nodes. He and his family knew that a melanoma like this was a very dangerous and potentially fatal cancer. He wanted to walk his daughter down the aisle for her wedding but the family was uncertain that he would be there for the event.

The treatment used against his cancer involved aggressive surgery, including the removal of the lymph nodes as well as chemotherapy. The treatment lasted for many months. We also employed experimental immunotherapy using cancer cells removed from his body at surgery to create a vaccine to inoculate him against his cancer. Several decades later, he still has no recurrence of the cancer and has not developed a new cancer. I do not know which of the treatments, other than the obvious role of the surgery, was critical to his survivorship. I suspect it was the immunotherapy, as we had been using the same chemotherapy on other patients with similar cancer for years without great long-term results, although it might have been good luck. The individual characteristics of this patient's cancer likely also played an important role in his good outcome. There were features of ongoing immune response seen in the lymph nodes that were removed at surgery.

The course of treatment for this patient was long and difficult. He became quite ill during the time of each chemotherapy treatment. His family, based on the advice from a relative who was an academic pathologist at a leading European medical school, did not want the lymph nodes removed. The family thought that such a procedure would weaken his immune system and would increase the chance of future spread and growth of the cancer.

In the end, despite his family's fear and uncertainty, my friend decided on the course of treatment that I advised. He walked his daughter down the aisle on her wedding day. Now our visits are focused on cancer survivorship. The risk of a cancer recurrence for this patient has declined after so many years, but is not zero. He is checked regularly for the development of any worrisome skin change that might suggest a new skin cancer. Advice is given regarding the prevention and treatment of other health issues that are common to cancer survivors, including screening for a new or recurrent cancers as well as for cardiovascular disease. Although he does not smoke and protects himself from the sun, exercise and a careful diet are additional steps for a healthy future.

The initial treatment of melanoma today would not differ from the treatment my friend received several decades ago. For recurrent melanoma there have been many advances. The cancer cells can now be evaluated for specific genetic changes that spur the growth of the cancer and this has led to new therapies that block the growth pathways. Newer immunotherapies have been developed that allow the patient's own immunosystem to overcome the blocks created by this cancer which allows the immune system to kill the malignant cells. This approach does not require the use of the patient's own cancer cells to create a vaccine. There is also a heightened awareness of the risk of developing melanoma which can lead individuals to extra vigilance, resulting in early detection and removal with a conservative surgical procedure with a very low chance of recurrence.

I recently advised a patient and his wife that, because a decade had passed since diagnosis and treatment of his rare heart cancer, we could stop follow-up testing for recurrence and instead focus on survivorship care. They felt relieved that I was confident in the prognosis and that they would not to have to continue to anxiously await test results every few months.

This particular patient and his wife were personal friends. The patient had collapsed at home in the early morning while showering. The evaluation which began in the emergency room uncovered a large tumor in the left atrium of the heart which was blocking flow out of the heart. After stabilization, the patient underwent urgent heart surgery to remove the tumor. The surgery was successful in restoring good blood flow and the patient felt better. Unfortunately, all of the cancer could not be removed. The fear was that the remaining cancer would grow and possibly spread.

The prognosis was very uncertain. The recommendations that were given to the patient ranged from removal of the heart followed by a heart transplant to observation only, with the hope that better treatments would become available in the future when needed. I saw him in a physician's role after this point. There was no standard treatment available for his condition but there were some promising possibilities. His cancer cell type was angiosarcoma which is a cancer of the blood vessel like cells. The taxane class of chemotherapy drugs had recently shown some promise in treating this cell type. There was a skilled radiation oncologist nearby who gave an opinion of the risks of combining radiation therapy to the residual cancer site as part of the treatment regimen.

After much discussion and after calling other oncologists at several medical centers working with this type of cancer, the patient began a course of chemobiological therapy followed by focused radiation. He did very well over all, although fatigue and nausea were a constant issue. Happily, after a decade, not only has the cancer not returned, there have been no side effects from his aggressive treatment. His focus is on a bright future.

three

Thank You, Doc

One of my patients had multiple aggressive squamous cell carcinoma that had spread widely. For years his metastatic disease could be controlled with chemotherapy, immunotherapy, and radiation therapy. At a later point, however, the cancer grew into a nerve in the arm affecting his use of the arm and causing him severe unrelenting pain. The surgeon suggested amputation to relieve the symptoms. The patient enjoyed his life and his family and was otherwise fairly fit. He had continued working throughout this difficult time. After full consideration, he chose to go forward with the amputation. This patient was able to cope very well, both physically and emotionally, with the loss of his arm. He continued to live a full life for a meaningful period of time.

Sometimes very aggressive treatment such as amputation can provide long-term relief from suffering. However, providing continuing care when the cancer cannot be cured remains an important part of an oncologist's work and is one of the most difficult roles the oncologist must fill. It is important to know when aggressive cancer treatment is more likely to harm than help. The thoughtful physician must consider when to change the focus to comfort care as the next story illustrates.

"Thank you, Doc. You were so good to us. Most importantly, you never said that there was nothing else to do." Hearing these words not long ago reminded me how I am always caught by surprise when a family member of a patient who has died comes to thank me. A patient's death always makes me feel inadequate and I struggle with the feeling that I have failed the patient and the family.

On this occasion, my patient's husband, who was a minister with a large congregation, came by my office a few days after his wife died of pancreatic cancer. When I first saw her two years earlier, she had been newly diagnosed with advanced pancreatic cancer. She had been given a life expectancy of less than six months by her other doctors. With aggressive chemotherapy, however, she dramatically improved and thrived for almost two years. Her cancer shrank to levels that could not be detected.

This woman was smart, funny, and full of life. She always had very strong opinions about her treatment. She told me to push forward as the treatment helped and when side effects of her treatment required a break, she was quick to advise. She first became aware of her cancer when she developed loss of appetite, weight loss, and abdomen pain. Tumors were found on a CT scan of her abdomen. A biopsy of the tumor using a thin needle guided by a CT scan image confirmed the diagnoses. She and her family were understandably frightened by the diagnosis and were distressed by her loss of appetite and weight loss. These manifestations of cancer can often dominate the discussion of cancer and are often a continuing source of worry, particularly for the family.

In the beginning of the journey, we talked about the nature of the cancer and how it caused her pain, loss of appetite, and weight loss. We talked honestly and openly about what could be done to help her. Pain control was critical and was the immediate focus. Although her cancer was very advanced and not curable, treatment could lead to improvement in her symptoms, particularly the pain and loss of appetite.

I held the cautious hope that she could continue her busy and productive life for some meaningful time. She knew a lot about cancer through her work in her husband's church. She wanted to get better but not be so ill from her treatment that she could not continue to be a part of her family and church life. She knew that this stage of pancreatic cancer could not be cured with the treatments available at the time and she never asked to be cured of the cancer.

When I first met this patient and her family, however, a new and promising treatment had been reported for pancreatic cancer. The medicine combination was complex to administer and had the potential of severe side effects. I discussed this new treatment with the patient and her family, with the hope that her cancer symptoms could improve if the cancer could be diminished in size. I thought that her overall health was good enough that the treatment could reasonably be prescribed if she wanted to undergo the experimental protocol.

Remarkably, she improved after the first treatment and was able to fully resume her life. The cancer greatly decreased in size. Further functional testing of the residual tumor found no activity using PET scanning, which is a measure of the metabolic activity of the tumor.

Side effects, however, did develop and after about nine months the treatment had to be stopped. After she recovered from the side effects, she felt well and decided that she wanted to put off any additional cancer treatments. She continued to be well for almost two years before she started to lose weight once again. Imaging studies confirmed a regrowth of the tumors. At her request and supported by her family, we began treatment again, but the side effects were such that she was better without active cancer treatment.

It was now time to consider her care going forward to allow her to be with those she loved and not undergoing debilitating treatment or in the hospital. We discussed at length focusing on treating her symptoms in her home with the help of hospice service, allowing me to continue to care for her. With medicines administered to her at home, she was able to remain a vibrant part of her family, until her heath. We continued medical therapy in the form of symptom management. Pain control remained the major focus. She continued with her active life which helped her maintain her good spirits and energy. Although her cancer caused fluid to build up in her abdomen which caused discomfort, I was able to remove the fluid on several occasions by draining it off with a needle. This simple outpatient procedure kept her comfortable.

The patient, her family, and I kept in close contact with visits and frequent phone calls. We always talked about how we would together continue to care for her. Hospice care was a continuation of that treatment with her goal of continuing in the life of her family and her church. She was at home when she died. Her family was gathered together around her and she was at peace.

Her husband was the first to call me to let me know of his wife's death. He and his family were grieving of course, but were together and looking to the future, knowing that they had done what they thought was right and feeling blessed that their wife and mother had lived for so long and that she had been able to continue to connect with her family and her church.

When her husband stopped by my office shortly after her death, he stressed how important it was that she had not been discharged from my care after active cancer treatment stopped and that I had never told her that there was nothing else to do for her. He told me stories of church members who had been abruptly told that there was nothing else to do for them and were discharged to the care of strangers. This was devastating to both the patients and their families. These stories surprised and saddened me.

I have learned that reassuring patients and their families that you will be available to them, and especially to help them with ongoing test and follow-up care, is of critical importance. Patients and families tell me that this is one of the most important points of providing effective cancer care. This commitment to an ongoing connection with the patient and family is what is meant in never saying that there is nothing else to do. The steady presence of the cancer doctor throughout the journey, including when the cancer is incurable, minimizes the fear and contributes to the well-being of both the patient and the family. This is a critical role of the oncologist as a doctor and as a human being.

four

The Early Years

The first meaningful advances in cancer treatment were marked by the early successes in treating acute leukemia followed by the treatment of lymphoma. Surgery had been the mainstay of cancer treatment for centuries. Too often the treatment came later and often the cancer recurred. Radiation therapy was then used in the late 19th century and again the same problems were observed. The first meaningful medical treatments using chemotherapy began in the late 1940's. Major advances were made when drugs were combined as had been done in treating tuberculosis using multiple drugs together.

The very earliest successful chemotherapy drugs were used in the treatment of leukemia and lymphoma. Acute leukemia is a dangerous blood disease usually found after the patient is suffering with fever and bleeding. It is a cancer that progresses quickly. These earliest drugs could reverse the situation for only a short time. When I was training in the field of hematology and oncology, there was still a debate about whether the use of any cancer treatment in adult leukemia was appropriate since the treatments were effective only in a small percentage of patients, the toxicities were great and the time of improvement was short and death inevitable.

Although progress in adult acute leukemia has improved, advances in children and young adult acute leukemias are even greater than in the adult acute leukemias. The most common subtype in adults is acute myeloid leukemia. This is in contrast to childhood and young adult leukemia where the most common subtype is acute lymphoblastic leukemia. The reasons for the current differences in outcome are not fully known. The adult acute leukemias have more acquired genetic changes and are more resistant to therapy. Adults who go into remission with chemotherapy, if fit enough, are often treated with additional high doses of chemotherapy and blood stem cell transplant because the outcomes are poor with chemotherapy alone. The treatments are very toxic. However, advances are being made.

One of the most dramatic and previously highly fatal form of acute myeloid leukemia is acute progranulocytic leukemia. The unusual complications of this form of the disease are due to the release of enzymes from the leukemia cells which destroy the blood clotting system leading to uncontrolled and fatal bleeding in a process called disseminated intravascular coagulation.

The genetic basis of this disease is now known to be chromosomal breakage with movement of a part of one chromosome to another chromosome creating a fusion gene that produces an abnormal retinoic acid receptor. Successful modification of this disease with a medicine called trans retinoic acid (ATRA), which modifies the abnormal gene product, quickly stops the bleeding and causes the leukemia cells to mature and then die. A newer drug derived from the chemical arsenic, called arsenic triode (ATO), is an effective treatment. Arsenic is a potentially dangerous poison but with a long history of use in medicine. When ATO is combined with ATRA, many patients are cured without the need for any chemotherapy or bone marrow or blood stem cell transplantation. This is one of the most remarkable stories in all of medicine.

Many patients undergo allogeneic bone marrow also known as stem cell transplantation as part of their therapy. The patient must be fairly fit and relatively young to qualify for the procedure. Allogeneic means the transplanted stem cells or bone marrow cells come from a donor as opposed to an auto transplant where the cells used are obtained from the patient. The benefit of allogeneic transplant appears to come from the immune system generated by the graft with the new immune cells, particularly lymphocytes, directly attacking any remaining leukemia cells. However, this immune attack, which is a form of immunotherapy, can become unregulated and cause graft versus host disease, which can lead to organ failure, infection, autoimmune disease and second cancer which are the great risks now of this procedure. The drugs most commonly used with the transplants can also cause infertility. Modification of the technique using low intensity induction holds the promise of successful treatment for older patients. Insights into the genetic basis of the leukemias is leading to new targeted therapies that are potentially more effective and safer. The auto-transplant depends on the availability of effective high dose drug therapy to kill the cancer with the reinfused stem cells, serving to minimize the toxic effects of the drug treatments on the blood cells.

Second cancers are a risk of many cancer therapies including stem cell treatments. A young woman was referred to me for treatment of abnormal blood counts found by her doctor when she saw him for weakness. She had delivered her first child only two months before. Her diagnosis was acute myeloid leukemia. She went into remission with chemotherapy and, because of the risk factors associated with her leukemia, she underwent an allogeneic stem cell transplant with cells from her brother. Although this patient developed a graft versus host disease, it appeared to mainly affect her skin. She was able to raise her child and carry on with her life for many years until she developed a rapidly growing and treatment resistant cancer of the tongue. This second cancer was a direct result of the graft versus host disease from her prior transplant. Although the leukemia never returned, the long term result was fatal to this wonderful young woman. Even at the end, she was grateful for the years she had with her adored child.

A happier outcome occurred for a young woman who also had undergone an allogeneic blood stem cell transplantation after a course of chemotherapy and an auto transplant, the full combination called a tandem transplant, for a recurrence of an aggressive Hodgkin's lymphoma. This patient doctor told her that she would be infertile from the treatment even though her treatment used a different set of chemotherapeutic drugs and a reduced intensity transplant. She never thought that she could conceive but to her great surprise and joy, she had a healthy son eight years after her treatment. When she came to see me so many years later she was afraid that her cancer had returned because she was vomiting and felt fatigue. How thrilled she was to learn that she was pregnant and cancer free.

The treatment of the chronic leukemias is also improving. Chronic lymphocytic leukemia is the most common of the adult leukemias. New chemotherapy drugs, immunotherapy drugs, and small molecule targeted therapies against over active cell growth pathways in the disease have extended life for many patients. Analysis of the genetic changes in the leukemia cells can even predict which patients will need treatment relatively soon as opposed to those patients that might not need treatment for decades, if ever. Sometimes, however, even patients with well controlled chronic lymphocytic leukemia can develop an aggressive cancer late in the course of the disease called a Richter's transformation which is the development of an aggressive and often treatment resistant lymphoma, arising out of the initial leukemia.

Another common form of chronic leukemia is chronic myeloid leukemia. This disease can be fatal in its own right but death usually comes when it progresses to an acute form of leukemia called a blast crises. This disease is often the result of an acquired genetic change in a blood cell precursor in the bone marrow that results in the transfer of genetic material from chromosome 9 to chromosome 21 called the Philadelphia chromosome. This was the form of acute leukemia that caused the death of the young woman from Wisconsin who loved the Green Bay Packers.

Today there are oral drugs that can block the cancer causing activity of mutated genes that cause this and other cancers. The results are so spectacular that most patients may never need any other therapy and traumatic outcomes such as occurred on the transplant ward when I was first in training may one day be a thing of the past.

The myelodysplasias (MDS) are a collection of pre-leukemia diseases most often seen in adults after the age of fifty. MDS can cause abnormal blood counts or an enlarged spleen. A high percentage of MDS patients ultimately develop acute leukemia. Patients who are young and healthy can be treated with acute leukemia-like drug regimens and an allogeneic blood stem cell transplantation. One advance are drugs that can change the genes expressed in the abnormal blood cells by modifying compounds that bind to the genes. This field of study, called epigenetics, holds promise for treating many other types of cancers as well.

I recall two patients whose blood diseases, although different, bridged two generations and two families. Both patients suffered from very low blood counts. One was an older man who was sent to me for low blood counts and an enlarged spleen. Despite these abnormalities, he felt well and his disease had, at first, little impact on his day to day life. Over the course of several years, he required occasional blood cell transfusions to maintain adequate hemoglobin to keep him functioning on a high level. During one of his visit to my office, he met another of my patients, a very young girl who suffered from severe aplastic anemia. This disease is a bone marrow failure disorder causing blood counts to fall to dangerously low levels. Low blood counts can lead to weakness when the red cell count drops to very low levels; bleeding can occur when the platelets drop to very low levels; and, infection can develop when the white blood cell count is very low, just as occurs in myelodysplastic. Often, this disease is due to an autoimmune attack where the patient's own immune system attacks the developing bone marrow cells, destroying the cells and preventing maturation into normal blood cells. This cancer can now be successfully treated by immunosuppressive therapy to inhibit the immune attack, sometimes requiring blood stem cell transplant combined with immunosuppressive therapy.

The young patient responded partly to the immunosuppressive therapy which improved her blood counts to a moderate degree, enough to keep her well for a time, but she ultimately succumbed to the disease. She had no donors to provide for an allogeneic stem cell transplant. Today, there are techniques for transplanting patients from unrelated or only partially matched donors or from placental blood cord blood which enlarges the pool of potential donors. At the time, however, the advances in treatment were years away.

The patient with myelodysplasia bonded with the little girl with aplastic anemia and became active in raising funds to help with the cost of her care. Even as he began to decline from the progression of his own blood disease, he continued his efforts for her. He told me that he believed it was far more important to help this young patient than focus on himself. He did not slow down his efforts despite his increasing disabilities including weakness, bruising and infection.

One day shortly before she died, my young patient proudly presented me with a baseball medal that she had won at a time when she was well. I still cherish this memento of her short but meaningful and positive life. She was an inspiration to others and loved by many.

Some patients with myelodysplasia do not need aggressive treatment since the risk of death from the treatments, particularly in older patients who are not well, is very high, and many can live well for a long time with supportive therapies such as transfusion of blood products. An older patient of mine had done well for years treated only with occasional transfusions. On a trip to his hometown to visit relatives, however, he was talked into a second opinion at the city's medical center. The doctor there recommended aggressive chemotherapy. The patient underwent the treatment and soon died of complications. He likely would have lived longer and with a good quality of life had he stayed with a supportive approach.

Treatment of all cancer types continues to advance. For the patients who came before, we are grateful to have helped them as best we could, balancing treatment with quality of life. To the patients now, the future holds great promise and hope.

five

Turning The Tide

During my time as a doctor, cancer death rates have markedly declined in the United States. This is true despite the overall increase in the number of cancers diagnosed, due in large part to the increasing number of older people in the population. In general, the risk of cancer increases with aging. Although in some parts of the world cancer deaths are rising, likely due to increased smoking and environmental toxicity, for the most part, the United States has seen an improvement not only because of our increased awareness of risk factors but also because of dramatic improvements in cancer treatment.

For example, the most aggressive type of brain cancer is glioblastoma multiforme. Until recently, few patients lived beyond a year even with treatment and most died within six months. Now medicines that were previously used to treat other cancers have shown benefit when added to the traditional treatments of surgery and radiation therapy.

A dramatic example of improvement in survival is the case of a young police officer I cared for who was diagnosed with a large glioblastoma multiforme. He was rushed to the emergency room after suffering a seizure. Before I saw him, he had undergone brain surgery with partial removal of the cancer. Brain cancers are very vascular and are prone to heavy bleeding. The patient suffered a severe hemorrhage at the surgical site the day after surgery. When I arrived for a consultation, he was unconscious and had no movement on his left side. He was on life support. His wife and children had been told that he had little to no chance of survival. The patient's extended family, who had gathered in the hallway, were shocked that this young man, who was perfectly well days before, was now near death.

With intensive care and some luck, the patient began to improve and was taken off life support. Although he remained paralyzed on his left side and had only half a normal field of vision because of the brain damage caused by the cancer and the hemorrhage, the patient was fully aware of his surroundings and could speak clearly. He and his wife hoped for a treatment that could provide him with a greater quality of life. Certain of his siblings, however, had no confidence in doctors or hospitals and advised that he be taken home without further treatment. Disagreement among family members occurs frequently, especially when the cancer type has a generally poor prognosis, and poses a particular problem for the cancer doctor. In this case, the wishes of the patient and his wife won the day and, over time, the rest of the family became more comfortable with choices made and with the treating doctors.

The treatment given to this patient was radiation therapy to the tumor combined with a chemotherapy pill and later a drug that inhibits tumor blood vessel growth that was first successfully used in colon cancer. Because the research was new, obtaining the drug for the brain cancer patient was difficult but ultimately successful. The patient had a stunning and long lasting shrinkage of the tumor. With his supportive family and rehabilitation efforts, the patient was able to live with some independence for six years before his cancer became resistant to further treatment. He passed away at home, in peace, surrounded by his family. I remember him as a strong and kind man who was blessed with a loving family. His story illustrates the great scientific advances that are made almost daily and that point to a brighter future for all cancer patients.

The amazing advances that continue to be made in our ability to treat cancer are due to incredible research that has increased our understanding of normal cell biology and what makes a normal cell cancerous. The journey to cancer wellness is marching forward; we are making dramatic progress in understanding and treating cancer. Even now there are tools available to study an individual person's cancer at the molecular level. This has already led to important changes in the way we understand and treat certain cancers.

We have learned that what earlier might have been simply an organ based cancer type such as leukemia, melanoma, kidney cancer, lung or breast cancer is instead unique to the individual suffering from the disease. The genetic and therefore the molecular characteristics often vary from one individual to another. It is no longer sufficient to make a diagnosis of cancer based on the organ of origin. We must personalize cancer treatment to the individual and that person's individual cancer.

At its root, cancer results from changes in the genetic material of a cell. These can be either changes in the genes themselves or changes that modify the activity of a gene, which is called epigenetics. One person's lung cancer is different from another person's lung cancer because of different combinations of genetic mutations. There mutations present unique targets for treatment. The breakthrough human genome project has opened the window on the cause of cancer.

Where do these genetic changes come from? Predisposition to cancer can be due to the inheritance of predisposing genetic changes that can be expressed anytime in life or acquired over time by environmental exposure such as cigarette smoking and radiation exposure. In some cases, it is a combination of these risk factors. Knowledge of the presence of these genetic changes may lead to effective preventative therapies to reduce the risk of subsequent cancer.

The inherited breast cancer gene mutations BRCA-1 and BRCA-2 increase markedly the risk for breast cancer, ovarian cancer, and other cancers in families that have these mutations. There inherited mutations cause about five percent of breast cancers. Screening for these mutations in families considered to be at high risk for carrying cancer causing genes has been demonstrated to be effective because the risk of developing cancer can be modified by surgical or medical methods. Individuals with the mutated familial adenomatous polyposis gene (FAP), which can cause colon cancer, can undergo preventative surgical treatment which is very effective in preventing the development of these cancers. The surgery to prevent breast cancer and ovarian cancer in carriers of BRCA-1 and 2 genes consists of removing the ovaries and adjacent structures before the age of fifty with possibly better success by the age of forty. The surgery for FAP includes removal of the colon and occasionally the rectum. We have not yet learned how to change the inherited genes at the genetic level to prevent these cancers. Perhaps preventative drug therapy or interventions to modify the effect of these abnormal cancer causing genes will soon be available.

The advances in our understanding of the genetic basis of cancer such BRCA and FAP abnormal genes lead to difficult decisions for the patient to minimize the risk of cancer development. The oncologist must be sensitive to patients' fears of testing and acting on results and help patients and their families in a guilt free and compassionate way.

I recall a young man I saw years ago with advanced colon cancer. He had hundreds of colon polyps identified early; he had inherited the abnormal FAP gene. Previous doctors had recommended enhanced screening with colonoscopy to remove the polyps and also recommended surgical removal of the colon as a more effective way to prevent cancer. For a number of reasons, primarily his fear of surgery, the patient did not follow this advice. He subsequently developed advanced colon cancer that was not curable.

Most mutations that cause cancer are not inherited but are acquired for reasons that are not clearly understood. An example is the mutated and over expressed HER-2 gene. This is not an inherited disorder but is acquired by the cell during its malignant transformation. In the past, finding this altered or over expressed gene in a breast cancer meant the outcome would be worse than average. Today, however, with this remarkable discovery, medical science has developed man-made antibodies and other drugs to inhibit the altered gene product, greatly improving the prognosis for affected patients. This discovery has been one of the most dramatic advances in breast cancer treatment.

Patients with lung cancer occasionally can also have effective gene directed treatment based on a specific mutation in the cancer cell's epidermal growth factor receptor which occurs in approximately 20% of lung cancer patients during cancer development but is more frequent in certain subsets of lung cancer particularly adenocarcenoma of the lung especially when the patient is female and a non smoker. The treatment utilizes medication that targets the specific gene product. Such treatment can avoid the toxicity of chemotherapy and provide better results.

A few years ago, I saw a woman with far advanced lung cancer who sought a second opinion regarding her cancer treatment. She had been treated for a year with surgery, radiation and chemotherapy for what was now a very far advanced lung cancer. I noted that she had not been evaluated for any of the recognized genetic mutations that can occur in lung cancer. We found a specimen of her tumor that had been removed several years before and stored. The cancer was an adenocarcinoma and she had never smoked. We analyzed the specimen for genetic mutations including the epidermal growth factor reception mutation. The test demonstrated the mutation. She was started on a daily pill to block the receptor, and she underwent dramatic improvement, with complete shrinkage of the tumor. She was able to live a full life without evidence of cancer for years. The ability to evaluate every patient's cancer cells for unique targetable genetic mutations at this individual level will continue to lead to treatment breakthroughs.

For some individuals, their cancer is clearly related to environmental factors. Smoking is one of the greatest disease causing agents of the modern world. Smokers have increased rates of heart disease and lung disease as well as cancer. It is relatively rare for a non-smoker to develop lung cancer. Studies have shown that if a person stops smoking, the risk of developing lung cancer declines shortly thereafter and falls to the risk level of a nonsmoker after twenty years of nonsmoking.

There are also environmental risks of developing breast cancer. For example, the incidence of breast cancer fell dramatically in this country after doctors curtailed prescribing estrogen and progesterone hormone replacement therapy to postmenopausal women. This has been difficult for many women because of the benefits of hormone replacement therapy for treating hot flashes and sweats. Ongoing research may allow for some forms of estrogen to be given without increasing the risk of cancer.

It is also now clear that our diet, weight, and our degree of physical activity impacts our risk of cancer. Being markedly overweight, in addition to causing other health issues like diabetes and heart disease, may play a role in the development of cancer development as well as the risk of recurrence after initial cancer treatment. There has been a lot of interest in using vitamins and other supplements to prevent cancer and there has been some evidence that a once-a-day multivitamin can increase life expectancy in part by decreasing the risk of developing cancer. Newer but incomplete evidence casts some doubt on the value of vitamins and supplements in prolonging life but this is still being studied. However, studies using specific vitamins such as C, E and betacarotene have not shown benefit and in fact may have caused harm.

My patients would agree that exercise, particularly walking or focused exercise such as yoga or Pilates, make them feel better. When they exercise, they have more energy, sleep better, and eat better. I believe it makes them healthier and decreases their risk of additional cancers. Exercise can be especially helpful during the period after active cancer treatment. There is strong evidence that regular exercise improves the quality of life, reduces the risk or a cancer recurrence and may reduce the risk of a new cancer developing.

Patients sometimes tell me that they are too tired to exercise. Fatigue is a symptom of cancer and cancer treatment. Paradoxically, however, exercising actually decreases the tired feeling. For patients who cannot get out and walk briskly for twenty minutes three of more times a week, I recommend swimming or exercising at home on a treadmill. With a CD or other video device, yoga or Pilates can be done at home on the patient's own schedule.

For years, a goal of medicine has been to find cancers early or to find precursor tumors that can be removed before cancer developed. Mammograms to detect breast cancer is a prominent type of screening. Some scientific institutes, however, have begun to debate the value of mammograms. Studies have also cast doubt on the benefit of prostate screening tests (PSA) for men. In truth, studies to date have shown very little mortality benefit derived from these tests. The cost to perform these tests in the United States is enormous and most observers agree that some harm can come from these tests. For example, most of the suspicious abnormalities seen on mammography are benign or of uncertain risk. In prostate cancer, there are many biopsies that show only low risk cancer. Patients then undergo subsequent procedures that can cause harm that may not be offset by any meaningful gain. Better tests performed on high risk individuals may be the answer in the future. The good news remains that breast cancer deaths in the United States have declined. Unfortunately, prostate cancer deaths remain unchanged.

To date, no screening tests are effective in detecting ovarian cancer. Many women have an increased risk for ovarian cancer, generally because of family history or inheritance of genes that can increase the risk for this cancer such as BRCA-1 and BRCA-2. These are the genes that also increase the risk for cancer.

Colonoscopy screening to remove polyps does seem to save lives. It may be that colonoscopy is a better test than mammography or PSA in detecting a meaningful abnormality. Also low dose radiation CT scans of the chest performed on individuals with a long history of tobacco use and a high lung cancer risk use can also detect some lung cancers at an early operable stage. However, as with mammography, many of the abnormalities prove to be benign.

Skin cancer screening is effective. The success of this test is probably because there is a direct observation of the area and the sites are easy and safe to biopsy. This holds for the common squamous cell and basal cell cancers of the skin as well as malignant melanoma.

Prostate cancer screening is complicated by continuing debate as to what to do once the cancer is found. Generally, the prostate cancer specialist will recommend treatment right away with either surgery, using either traditional or robotic techniques, or radiation called brachytherapy using radioactive material placed directly into the prostate gland during a minor surgical procedure if the cancer is small and localized. Sometimes, watchful waiting is recommended, particularly if the patient is over seventy-five or in poor health. The reason not to treat immediately is because for some low grade cancers, the behavior is uncertain. There are also risks from the treatment, including erectile dysfunction, urine or bowel difficulties.

Watchful waiting is effective when warranted but requires regular medical evaluation over many years. I treated a patient with advanced prostate cancer that developed six years after he was found to have an intermediate risk prostate cancer based upon a high PSA level found at a yearly health physical. He was in his late seventies at diagnosis and he was in his early eighties when I saw him. He was in quite poor health overall. The prostate cancer had spread to his bones when I saw him. He expressed anger that his first doctor had not pushed him to have treatment at the time of his initial diagnosis. What he did not appreciate was that while he had chosen watchful waiting, he had failed to have regular checkups, which may have found the aggressive change in his cancer before it spread and allowed for effective treatment. For this patient, both his cancer and symptoms were able to be controlled for many more years but he did not die of old age, rather, he died from this prostate cancer many years after the initial diagnosis.

It is quite likely that in the next few years it will be routine to study an individual's genetic makeup as part of a routine health evaluation such as is done for hypertension and hyper chloresterolemia. The analysis of the genetic changes will lead to prevention, early diagnosis and, when needed, effective therapy. This will be the best preventive screening.

We are in an era of dramatic advances in our understanding and treatment of cancer. We still have some distance to go but the path ahead is clear. One day we will prevent most cancers and others will be successfully treated.

six

Cancer In The Young

There were occasions early in my career when I treated children and young adults. The reasons varied, but for the most part this was because the young patients and their families could not travel to obtain care at a distant medical center. The common impression is that treating children or young adults with cancer is especially difficult for a doctor, but that is not necessarily the case. Children with cancer are incredibly brave, open, and honest. Their main focus in not on themselves; they worry about their parents and siblings and how cancer will affect them. Further, in terms of outcome, children and young adults treated appropriately generally have good outcomes, although not always.

The most common cancer in both children and adolescents are blood related cancers of leukemia and lymphoma. For children, cancers of the nervous system, that is, brain, nerves and supporting structures, represent a large percentage of cancers. Children also tend to have more sarcomas than adults. Sarcomas are cancers of the supporting structures of the body such as bones and cartilage. Adolescent cancer seems to fall between children and adult cancer. Adolescents with leukemia have better outcomes when treated with therapies that copy the very successful childhood leukemia regimens which are marked by higher drug doses and more frequent dosing of two drugs, vincristine and asparaginase. It is remarkable that improvements in treating acute lymphoblastic leukemia is through the use of older drug in new ways rather than new drug discoveries.

Many years ago, a local pediatric oncologist called me to say that he was closing his practice to begin training in psychiatry. He had several patients who were not able or willing to leave town for treatment. He asked if I would see these young patients and I agreed. The care of these patients enriched my life.

One of the young patients sent to my care was a teenager with advanced and progressing sarcoma that had first developed in the tissue surrounding a shoulder joint. She had been treated with surgery, radiation, and chemotherapy with transient benefit and was now failing. Through it all, she remained cheerful and upbeat. She told me she had to keep positive and had to keep trying to live for her parents' sake. She did not want to cause them pain and sorrow.

She responded well for about a year to a newly developed chemotherapy treatment. Although she lost her hair with the treatment, that did not bother her at all. Walking through the hospital one day, I passed several young girls all dressed up in elaborate costumes for Halloween. As I passed, one of the girls called out "Don't you recognize me with my hair?" My patient had on a shiny red wig and sparking costume to celebrate the holiday. She was as excited and energetic as her friends who had come to spend Halloween with her.

Her parents believed that vitamin supplements, and particularly that vitamin C in large doses, would help their child. Even near the end of her life, her father felt comforted by continuing to give her vitamins. I saw no harm in continuing this for his daughter and I cheerfully complied with her father's wishes. She never lost her sense of fun and her love of her family. The children and young adults who suffer with cancer are the strongest and most inspiring among us.

Not all sarcomas are high grade and aggressive in their behavior. In these cases, it is important to be thoughtful and avoid overtreatment in the young patient. A young man, who is now finishing his studies for the ministry, years ago found a lump in his upper thigh. It was painless and seemed to have come from nowhere. He had a wife and young children. He worked on the docks as a longshoreman and attended divinity school part time. A fine-needle biopsy

showed a soft tissue sarcoma, likely from the skeletal mus-
cle in the thigh. It is important to use a minimally invasive
technique when sarcoma is suspected because big biopsies
can make complete removal of the cancer difficult and can
increase the risk that the cancer will grow back in the same
location. Imaging studies with CAT and PET scans showed
no evidence of spread.

I advised removal of the cancer surgically with attention to
obtaining a margin of healthy tissue around the surgical specimen. Pathological studies on the resected cancer showed that
while the cancer was large, about 4.5 cm, it was low grade. I
recommended no further treatment such as chemotherapy or
radiation therapy because the risk of the adjuvant treatments
outweighed the benefit because his cancer had a low chance of
recurrence or spread to other parts of this body. This young
man has remained healthy and he was happy that he was not
talked into more toxic treatments. He will soon finish his training as a minister and I have no doubt that he will have a big
congregation and will provide comfort and joy to many.

The diagnosis of cancer in a young person is achingly sad
for the family. The distress can be acutely felt and readily
understood, whether the patient is a child or a young adult.
It always amazes me how brave these young patients are and,
after a period of time, how well their families begin to deal with
this most difficult situation.

It is in this context that I remember a young man with Down's syndrome and acute leukemia, brought to me by his parents for diagnosis and treatment. The family wanted him to be treated near home, because they thought that neither he nor they would do well at a large academic medical center. Children with Downs syndrome are known to have an increased risk of leukemia, and the leukemia tends to be more aggressive than that in other children and young adults. Fortunately, this patient had an excellent response to treatment, and his leukemia went into remission.

The treatment, consisting of intravenous injection therapy, was difficult and complex. With the active support of his family, the young patient took all the interventions in stride. The most difficult days were those on which a bone marrow biopsy or spinal tap needed to be performed. Bone marrow biopsies done with a special needle on a pelvic bone were needed to determine the status of the leukemia. The spinal taps were needed to check for leukemia cells in that area, as well as to administer chemotherapy directly into the spinal fluid.

These procedures are easier for all if the patient is able to remain still for a brief period of time. In this case, the patient's brother, a former wrestler, would come into the room to help keep the patient in position. His presence was always calming. Talking to the young patient during the procedure also helped. The preparation for the procedure was a joint effort on the part of all involved. The patient would let me know when it was all right to proceed by saying "Ok, I'm ready," and the procedure would then go forward. To prevent postprocedure headaches after spinal taps, I suggested he drink a can of Mountain Dew, a soft drink with caffeine, and I would drink a can with him. After the procedure, his family would take him for lunch. He looked forward to the ritual and these treats made procedure days much less fearful.

This young patient loved to do art work and would often bring me his work to review and express my delight and praise. In fact, his work was quite good. As a keepsake for my desk, he painted a smiling face on a rock. I still have his gift.

Pediatric hematologists were once known as the angels of death because of the very poor prognosis for young patients in the early days of cancer treatment. This is no longer true. Great strides have been made in curing the cancer of young people. The cure rate is so high that there can now be efforts made to reduce the intensity of treatment for some in order to decrease the risk of toxic effects and serious late effects such as second cancers, growth and developmental abnormalities, and reductions in fertility so that these young patients can look forward to a full and happy life.

Preserving fertility for children and young adults is a challenging issue that is finally receiving attention. Oncologists, patients, and families need to consider the effects of cancer treatment on the subsequent ability of the young patient to have children. Safer treatments at less intense levels will continue to play a positive role. For other situations, the family should consider preemptive sperm or egg retrieval and storage for later assisted reproduction, if needed. There are organizations that exist to assist in this matter.

A few years ago a former patient of mine, who had survived advanced testicular cancer as a child, came to me for a checkup. I had not seen him for several years. Although there was no sign of his cancer, it was clear that he had not been taking good care of his health. He worked full time and did not exercise, his diet was poor, and he smoked heavily. His cholesterol was high. He told me that he was soon to marry.

I took the opportunity to focus this young man on the need for a healthier life. He stopped smoking, started exercising, and ate better. He took a cholesterol-lowering medicine to bring his levels to a safe number. We talked about his ability to father children. At the time, he was not able to have children naturally because the surgery he had undergone to remove residual abdominal masses that had persisted after his chemotherapy had damaged the nerves controlling sperm ejaculation. I then talked with the patient and his new wife about possibilities. I advised that he undergo sperm retrieval by performing a small biopsy of his healthy testicle. This was successful and a happy, healthy child was born using assisted reproduction. The couple plan more children in the future.

Childhood cancer generally has a good outcome. To take advantage of the advances in pediatric and young adult cancers, I cannot overemphasize the need for expert care utilizing second opinions where appropriate. Actions should be taken promptly. Delay in treatment, particularly for childhood leukemia and lymphomas, can be dangerous. Of course, treatment is not always successful. Patients and their families need advice and counsel should end of life issues arise. I have been to funerals of young patients and I am always inspired by the strength of the survivors.

An example of the success of new treatments is the story of the young man who came in recently for a checkup. He was three years out from the time of his diagnosis of multiple myeloma. He was a teenager when the diagnosis was made. He had been ill for a year with severe generalized bone pain. His initial doctors could not establish a cause for his pain. He had scarring changes in almost all of his bones that, in retrospect, was highly suspicious for multiple myeloma. His doctors did not further explore this in detail, however, because he was so young and appeared otherwise healthy. They did not consider a cancer diagnosis likely. Finally, a biopsy of the bone was done using a needle guided by a CT scanner. The family was told of the diagnosis during a late night phone call from these doctors. Emergency referral to a distant medical center was urgently advised. Friends of the mother saw her misery and suggested that they see me for a second opinion.

The distress in the patient and family was understandably severe. They feared that the late diagnosis might negatively affect any treatment possibilities for this young man. To add to their misery, the patient's father had died unexpectedly the previous year from a heart attack.

In this case, treatment was extremely successful and was based on a program that used newly available medications. The patient did develop severe leg pain, which over time resolved. Today, he is active and looking forward to his life to come. Both he and his family are realistic about the chance for a cure and anxiety is quick to resurface, particularly during periods of retesting and waiting for the results of bone marrow biopsies and laboratory studies.

seven

Aftermath Of The Battle

The patient, in his late sixties, was having trouble swallowing again. Six months earlier, he had been treated successfully for a large squamous cell cancer of the esophagus. He smoked tobacco and drank alcohol in excess, all of which likely caused his cancer. This tumor had been high in the esophagus just below the throat. The location of the tumor meant that surgery was not an option because of the difficulty in recreating a swallowing tube after removal of that portion of the esophagus. The patient was treated with radiation combined with chemotherapy given at the same time over a seven week period.

The tumor was first discovered when the patient had trouble swallowing and felt throat pain. Treatment was successful and the cancer disappeared. Six months later, however, the patient noticed constriction in the treated area of the esophagus. This proved not to be a recurrence of cancer but the result of scar tissue forming from the radiation. Unfortunately, this is a common problem after radiation to that part of the body.

Treatment of this restriction, called stenosis, was successful and consisted of a series of dilations of the esophagus using tubes of increasing diameter passed through the area of stenosis during an upper esophageal endoscopy performed by a gastroenterologist. Light sedation was given and the process took only minutes at each treatment. It was repeated a few more times over a year. The procedure was successful and the patient's swallowing became normal again.

When the upper esophageal cancer was diagnosed, the patient was also evaluated for potential other cancers of the upper airway and esophagus that could be caused by smoking. He had a precancerous area on his vocal cord. This too went away with the radiation. In the meantime, the patient stopped smoking and cut back on his alcohol intake. There has been no new or recurrent cancer. This patient's cancer did not have to happen, however. It might not have occurred but for his cigarette smoking and excessive alcohol use.

Sometimes radiation therapy causes damage that does not reverse itself or is too severe to be repaired. I was asked to care for a young man whose in-laws were my patients. Although he never smoked cigarettes, he did smoke marijuana on a daily basis. He had developed a large tumor in the left side of his neck which originated from a tumor of the mouth which then spread to the lymph nodes in his neck. This young man had already dealt with more life challenges than most people many years his senior. He had first faced kidney cancer and had a kidney removed. Now he was faced with mouth and neck cancer. He would later develop and survive prostate cancer. His parents had survived the concentration camps of Europe during World War II, perhaps giving him the never give up attitude that remained with him throughout his cancer journey. His wife was loving and supportive which was a critical factor in helping him cope with so much adversity.

Several years after he was treated successfully for mouth and neck cancer, he began to have trouble swallowing. The radiation had damaged his swallowing muscles. Ultimately, he had to have a tube placed into his stomach through the abdominal wall, called a PEG tube, so that he could get nutrition. Why did this young man have so many cancers and why did he have such a severe reaction to radiation? The answers are not known but, one day, advances in the genetic basis of cancer will allow us to understand. Advances will also allow less toxic treatments and perhaps even prevent the cancers from developing in the first place.

Some cancers of the upper airway we now know are caused by chronic virus infection. The cancer causing virus is called the human papilloma virus and is acquired by exposure. This is the same virus that causes cancer of the cervix in women. It can also cause cancer of the anus and male penile cancer. Screening for cervical cancer with the Pap test performed by gynecologists during routine female health exams has decreased mortality for cervical cancer. Unfortunately, there currently exists no good screening for the other cancers caused by this virus.

Curiously, the virus caused cancers of the upper airway seem to have a better outcome with conventional therapy using surgery, radiation, chemotherapy, and immunotherapy that the nonviral caused cancers of the upper airway. Because of the advances in understanding the virus causing cervical cancer, we may be able to prevent these other human papilloma caused cancers. Cervical cancer can be prevented by vaccinating young girls against the virus. As a result, perhaps for the next generation, cervical cancer will disappear. Perhaps this vaccine will also prove effective in preventing other human papilloma virus caused cancers.

For many, the years following cancer treatment can be difficult because of the lasting effects of treatment as well as the risk for recurrence or new cancers. Years ago I saw a young woman who had just undergone surgery for pancreatic cancer. The cancer was too advanced to be removed. Before her diagnosis she had suffered with abdominal pain and developed jaundice, which is a yellow discoloration of the eyes and skin. With this she had developed very dark urine and almost white stools. The jaundice was due to elevated bilirubin in her skin and the urine and stool changes were from blockage of the bile ducts by the cancer preventing bile pigments from getting to the intestine for removal. As a consequence, it would build up in the blood and show up in the urine. Her doctor performed a CT scan initially and saw the large tumor and the blocked bile ducts.

This patient's tumor was too extensive to be removed surgically. However, she was able to undergo a surgical procedure that bypassed the blocked ducts by creating a new drainage tract using her intestine. She had an easy recovery from the surgery. Her jaundice disappeared because of the bypass of the bile duct blockage. Nevertheless, she began to lose weight and her abdominal pain persisted. She was told her future was very grim. She came to see me for any possible cancer treatment.

In those days, the treatment for a large pancreatic cancer that could not be removed consisted of radiation to the tumor given at the same time as intravenous administration of chemotherapy. The hope was that the chemotherapy would make the radiation treatment more effective. Radiation therapy by itself had only minimal beneficial effects and the chemotherapy alone was relatively ineffective. Today fortunately, chemotherapy and other measures are more effective.

Remarkably, the treatment this patient was given was very successful, and her cancer went away. She has been cancer free now for several decades. I would not have predicted such a happy outcome. Life for her was far from easy though. Her husband died of heart disease at a young age. Her mother, whom I treated, developed and survived breast cancer and non-Hodgkin's lymphoma only to die much later from yet another cancer. Her brother, who lived elsewhere, had kidney failure. Her sister developed lung cancer. My patient had to be the primary caregiver for her family as well as deal with the after effects of her own cancer.

She pushed herself to provide this needed care to others, all the while developing additional health problems for herself. Some of these issues were the result of her cancer treatment and some due to the development of new health problems that often occur in cancer survivors. She developed hypertension, high cholesterol, and diabetes. She developed a chronic fatigue and chronic pain syndrome. The treatment complications kept her from working. Health insurance was impossibly expensive for her because of her health history. She developed a sense of pervasive guilt that she had survived while her other family members did not. Too many cancer survivors have similar stories that blunt the joy of living after cancer.

Because of her financial and health insurance issues, which limited her access to traditional primary healthcare, I became her primary physician. We, together, have been able to address her health issues, and she is now doing much better. Chronic low energy remains, however, as does her chronic pain requiring ongoing treatment. There are also worries about new cancers, because of the multiple cancers in her family. Nevertheless, I am optimistic about her future. She has overcome an inordinate amount of hardship and she should be very proud of her accomplishment.

The success of modern cancer treatment means that there will be many more survivors of a cancer diagnosis and therefore many more people and their families developing these later cancer survivor problems. It is clear we need a major effort to develop the tools to identify these later health and survivorship problems. We also need better tools to prevent and treat these problems for both the patients and their families who are understandably stressed from the cancer diagnosis and potentially at risk for increased risk of future cancers. It has become clear to me that those involved in survivorship care must use new multifaceted approaches for both patients and their families to help them lead happy and fulfilling lives.

First, to have an honest and open exchange among the cancer caregiver, the patient, and the family about the cancer at hand and the anxiety the cancer causes can go a long way to improving the chances for successful cancer survivorship. I am often told that the initial interaction between the patient and the cancer doctor is too technical and clinical and often only adds to the stress level of the patient and family. The medical message is often unclear and future plans vague. The doctor must recognize that a sense of urgency verging on panic is the typical response after the cancer diagnosis.

Part of the problem in the relationship between the cancer patient and the doctor is that many physicians are personally very uncomfortable with issues of survivorship and death. Doctors tend to focus on matters they can control, such as the technical aspects of treatments and the timing of treatments. Patients and their families that I see after the initial cancer diagnosis and any initial surgical treatment often have little or no knowledge about subsequent treatment and issues of survivorship. For example, topics such as jaundice, the retention of the bile component bilirubin, that developed in my patient with advanced pancreatic cancer, can be bewildering.

Second, there needs to be an organized way for the cancer survivor to obtain appropriate and ongoing health counseling and care. Our current system remains too fragmented and for many far too difficult to access, allowing may health problems that are unique to the cancer survivor to be overlooked or not addressed in a timely manner.

eight

Continuing Vigilance

The questions of why me and how did this happen are always asked after a cancer diagnosis. We know that smoking and certain environmental exposures such as asbestos cause cancer. For most people with cancer, however, the triggering event is unknown.

Further, we do not yet know why a cancer that has been in remission for years or decades after treatment suddenly starts to regrow. This is often seen in breast cancer patients. Half of the recurrences of low-risk breast cancer that are destined to recur do so after five years, a time after which most patients think of themselves as cured. We know that the type of active treatment at the time of diagnosis, such as chemotherapy or endocrine therapy, does not prevent this late recurrence. Particularly with breast cancer, research is ongoing to find a better way to prevent late recurrence with either prolonged initial treatment or newer therapies still under investigation. Evidence suggests that ten years rather than the standard five years of adjuvant endocrine therapy may modestly decrease the risk of recurrence.

The best current thinking suggests that late recurrence may be due to previously quiescent cancer stem cells developing new genetic changes which allows growth resumption. Another possibility is that there has been a change in the local environment where that dormant cancer cell lives that stimulated regrowth. The concept that the local area microenvironment can regulate cancer cell growth is a new and promising area of cancer study and is illustrated in new treatments for multiple myeloma, a form of blood cancer.

Some new cancers discovered long after treatment of the initial cancer may be brought on by the same cause of the first cancer, such as smoking, but others may be the direct consequence of the otherwise effective treatment use to cure the initial cancer. Some chemotherapy drugs and radiation treatment can cause late development of myelodysplasia, which is a form of a malignant blood disease, acute leukemia, as well as solid organ based cancers such as sarcomas, which are cancers of the bone and other connecting tissues that hold organs in place. Other late effects of initial cancer treatments may include the development of heart disease, both heart attacks and heart failure, which present many years later. Some patients develop treatment caused memory loss that can be irreversible.

Oncologists are now aware of these late effects of cancer treatment. Survivorship care, that is, care after treatment, is a critical aspect of good cancer care. The thoughtful physician will discuss with the patient and family the issues and weigh the risk of late effects with the risk of not treating the cancer presented. Unfortunately, many patients and their families are not aware of the risks created by their cancer treatments. It should be a factor in the treatment decision making process. The need for a more formal follow-up survivorship program should be recognized and protocols developed.

Although it has been said that there is no measurable benefit to the traditional yearly heath checkup, focused checkups tailored to the cancer patient should yield measurable benefits. Other important issues that should be considered and treated in survivorship programs include those that may be experienced by young cancer patients. Children treated for cancer have an increased risk of learning disorders, behavioral problems, obesity, diabetes mellitus, hypertension, heart disease, as well as fertility. These findings have led to modifications in the initial cancer treatment of children and a recognition that follow-up care is important. Effective interventions exist and are under study to lower these risks to children with cancer.

An example of the issues presented in dealing with late effects from cancer treatment is illustrated by a young woman I cared for years after her initial diagnosis of breast cancer and treatment by another doctor. Eight years after her first breast cancer was diagnosed and treated, she was diagnosed with breast cancer in her other breast. In the interim, she had developed heart failure from the chemotherapy given in her initial treatment for her first cancer. She was a patient without any unusual risk factor for breast cancer, there were no exposures or a family history of breast cancer and she did not carry the known inherited breast cancer gene BRCA1 or BRCA2.

Her new breast cancer was successfully treated. Unfortunately, her heart condition worsened over time until her cardiologist advised her to accept hospice care with comfort measures only. Her doctor determined that because of her second cancer, despite remission, she was not a candidate for a heart transplant since transplant protocols keep a patient who has a recent diagnosis of cancer from transplant eligibility. She was told that nothing more could be done and that she would soon die.

When I saw this patient for a second opinion, there were new techniques that could serve as a bridge to heart transplantation or perhaps replace heart transplantation altogether. The former Vice President of the United States had just received an implanted left ventricular assist device to his failing heart and ultimately underwent a successful heart transplant. With this success in mind, I encouraged this young woman to consider such a ventricular assist device. She concurred and I found an academic medical center who agreed to perform the procedure. Today, this young woman is not only cancer free, but her heart condition is under control and she has returned to work.

It is not unusual to see an advanced cancer that could have been effectively treated had the patient sought medical care at an early stage. I have seen this most often in cases of breast cancer and colon cancer. The common explanation by the patient is fear of cancer and its treatment. All have the hope that the problem would just go away. A woman in her forties was referred to me by an emergency room physician. She had gone to the ER because of bleeding in her left breast. She had a large ulcerated cancer the size of an orange that had ruptured. The bleeding was from the raw surfaces of the ruptured site. Despite its advanced state, the cancer had not spread to other parts of her body. Chemotherapy, surgery with a mastectomy, and later radiation therapy and endocrine therapy put the patient into remission. After seven years, the cancer has not recurred. But how had the patient, who was a wife and mother, kept her cancer a secret for so long? She wore elaborate clothing to cover her tumor in order to prevent others from knowing about the growth. Her husband told me that he had no idea of the problem because of her ruses; he and his wife carried on a full married relationship, but he never knew about the tumor.

Ten years ago I treated a woman, then in her late seventies, who had also ignored a breast cancer for several years. She had developed bleeding which led to the diagnosis of cancer. Despite the delay, the cancer had not spread beyond the breast. This was not simply luck but more likely the genetic makeup of her cancer cells which had not yet undergone the genetic mutations leading to cancer spread. The molecular basis for cancer spread appears to be different from the mutations that initially cause a cancer. When diagnosed, this patient was not well enough for chemotherapy and surgery would have been very deforming. Further, she refused any surgery or chemotherapy. Her cancer, however, proved to be responsive to endocrine therapy directed at blocking the stimulating effect of her body's estrogen on the cancer cells. After a very dynamic response to the endocrine therapy, she was given radiation to her chest wall, lymph nodes, and breast. She tolerated the treatments very well and her cancer has not returned.

Several years into this patient's treatment, I was called by her daughter who had just received a diagnosis of rectal cancer after a colonoscopy. She had observed blood in her stool and rectal pain for over a year yet had told no one about her symptoms because, much like her mother, she feared the potential consequences of acknowledging her problem. She also felt she was too busy caring for her parents and her own family to acknowledge her own health issues.

A CT scan demonstrated that the cancer had spread to her liver. This young woman has done very well after aggressive treatments and, seven years after her initial diagnosis, is in good health and fully recovered. Despite her fears, with the success of her progressive treatment, she did not need extensive surgery which could have resulted in a colostomy, which is the stool diversion procedure which can be necessary if the cancer is too large or too low in the rectum. I referred her for surgery after her excellent response. She had only a few residual cancer cells at the rectal site. No remaining cancer was found in the liver.

My brother asked me to see the younger sibling of one of his childhood friends for an opinion on treatment of a recently diagnosed venous thrombosis which is a blood clot in a vein. The patient had pain and swelling in his leg. He went to the local emergency room for an evaluation and an ultrasound test on the leg revealed the blood clot. He was placed on blood thinning agents, call anticoagulants, to prevent the clot from enlarging or breaking off and moving to the lungs. His body's natural clot dissolving enzymes, in a process called fibrinolysis, destroyed the clot. He was placed on warfarin after initial and overlapping heparin therapy but experienced difficulty in establishing the correct dosing strength. After a short time, the patient's anticoagulation was under control.

The cause of the blood clots was still unknown. This patient had no known risk factors for blood clots. Some patients have a family history of blood clots and there are inherited factors that can explain the reason for blood clots. Other times, blood clots follow surgery because of limited mobility and the stimulation of the clotting system that can result from surgery. This patient, however, had not been immobilized or bed ridden. He had not taken any long flights or car trips. He was not taking any medication that could cause blood clots. He had no family history of blood clots. He was, however, over forty. Cancer is one of the more common causes of unprovoked deep venous thrombosis after a certain age. A CT scan of his abdomen showed a kidney cancer that likely predated the initial diagnosis by months or even a year. There was no sign that the cancer had spread. Nevertheless, the whole kidney had to be removed because the cancer was large and not positioned to allow for a partial kidney removal. The patient recovered and finished his course of blood thinner medications. He has remained cancer free.

Avoiding diagnosis and care because cancer is thought to be an enemy stronger than ourselves is a mistake. Self-awareness and taking steps for personal well-being are the foundations for prevention and cure. There is always hope and the rapid advances in treatment and quality of life are in the present. The strength that can be derived from a positive view of the future is a key to wellbeing. In my office waiting room, I always kept pale blue pebbles in a simple white bowl as decoration. The pebbles would disappear over time and new ones had to be found as replacements. I asked where they went and was told that some patients focused on the pebbles as a symbol of calm and good luck and would pocket one to keep at home as a positive force. Luck is less necessary today than before in the battle against cancer; calm and a positive view are still useful tools in the battle.

nine

Defeating The Enemy

A person diagnosed with cancer today has a very good chance of survival and cure. The prognosis for patients with cancer is improving at a rapid rate. Finding a highly skilled and empathetic doctor increases the chance of a good outcome. Each patient with cancer is distinct and individual and each patient's concerns are also unique. In all cases, prognosis, treatment and follow-up care must be personalized.

Years ago I met a patient who had just undergone an operation to remove a tumor that had developed in her lung. It was a recurrence of a kidney cancer that had been treated with kidney removal ten years before. A search for other sites of cancer spread showed several small tumors in the lung not seen before her lung surgery. Since that time, she had been given a sequence of modern targeted agents that did not include chemotherapy. Her cancer cells developed resistance to some treatment but second and subsequent generations of these treatments were developed and were successful for her. She had four treatment regimens. This patient remained well and active because of this breakthrough development in therapy, targeted to her individual specific cancer.

It is critical to promptly make the correct diagnosis, which directly leads to the best possible treatment. For rare cancers or for a cancer for which there is not a good treatment available, the best doctors will search for further information and allow a referral to a doctor or a cancer center elsewhere that might have promising experimental treatments.

It is very important that the cancer patient and family have a doctor or other advocate who is willing and committed to do the right thing for the patient and family. There must be a plan of action at the earliest phase of a cancer diagnosis. More preliminary tests may be necessary. My patients and their families have told me that they can feel paralyzed at this point. Even if told what the next steps are, they are not able to act alone. It is important that the advocate personally arrange for the next steps with all the details of tests, referrals, and information.

Several years ago, I was asked to see a young man who was brought to the emergency room minutes after he stepped off an airplane. He had come to visit his mother for the summer. She was alarmed the moment she saw him. He was weak and pale and admitted that he had been ill for over six months. He had noticed a lump in his scrotum and it had grown larger. He had little appetite, had lost almost fifty pounds and had developed some difficulty breathing.

His family doctor at home had concluded that an infection was the explanation for the enlarging scrotal tumor and had been treating him with antibiotics. Unfortunately, this was incorrect. The diagnosis was advanced testicular cancer. When I discussed this with the patient and his mother, they were understandably devastated. The tumor was the size of an orange. He also had orange-sized tumors in his lungs, which were causing breathing problems, and the same sized tumor in his abdomen.

The delay in diagnosis is what caused his overall health to become so poor. It may have been that the family doctor had little experience with testicular cancer and was simply focused on infections, as infections are a common problem seen by family practitioners. Human inclination is to avoid a frightening diagnosis, such as cancer, and this may have also have played a role. Perhaps a combination of such preconditions led to the delay.

I also emphasize to patients and families that they should push for re-evaluation and perhaps a second opinion if a medical situation continues to deteriorate in the face of treatment for a presumptive diagnosis. Fortunately, this young man had a very good response to treatment and returned to good health.

The ability to cure even advanced testicular cancer is one of the most remarkable achievements in oncology. The drugs now used to treat this disease became available in the 1970s and 80s. The drugs have side effects; nerve damage and lung damage as well as severe nausea and vomiting can result. However, the last ten years have seen major advances in preventing some of these side effects, especially vomiting. I recall when I was beginning my training at an international cancer center, I treated a young man who had testicular cancer. Effective treatment was just being developed and there was little we could do to prevent the terrible nausea and vomiting side effects caused by the new drugs. The young may would fly in from West Texas on a regular schedule for chemotherapy. He brought one suitcase with only his toothbrush, a change of clothes, and a bottle of Mescal, the liquor with the worm in the bottle. He hid the bottle from the nurses but he told me that drinking Mescal was the only way that he could get through the debilitating treatment.

Better outcomes in cancer treatment have been the case now for a number of years. For some cancers, effective chemotherapy treatment first developed several decades ago is still being used. For most cancers, treatment is not yet quite as successful as that for testicular cancer but is improving as we better understand the nature of cancers at the genetic level. Some cancers, which also include childhood acute lymphoblastic leukemia and Hodgkin's lymphoma, respond very well to chemotherapy treatments. The reason for this is not definitively known although it is likely due to the molecular basis of these cancers and a lack of resistance mechanisms. That said, even today the cure rates are not 100% for these cancers.

Childhood cancers in general tend to be more responsive to treatment than adult cancers. The reason again is not known, but I believe is a function of the less extensive genetic changes that lead to childhood cancer compared to the complex genetics of adult cancers. The outcome for adult cancers is improving, and there is no reason to doubt that improvements will accelerate because of our ability to now take a deep dive into the genetic changes in these cancers.

Scientists now have a clear goal in studying the genetic basis of individual cancers. After the advances made by the human genome project, it took years to analyze the genes of one human and cost millions of dollars. This analysis can now be done in days and soon perhaps in hours, and will be performed at a cost that will allow this deep sequencing dive to be available as a routine laboratory test on the same biopsy that is used to make the cancer diagnosis. Already, the identity of abnormal genes and their protein products can, for many cancers, be identified and simple corrective therapies given, often using pills rather than shots or injections.

What about preventing cancer in the first place? It is quite clear that the environment and individual behavior account for over half of all adult patients. Modifying these factors should decrease the number of patients who develop cancer. Tobacco smoking is leading environmental and behavioral cause of cancer. Individuals who stop smoking will decrease their risk for many cancers, not just lung cancer. These individuals will have a lower risk of heart attack and stroke. Regular exercise and weight control also have a real effect in reducing cancer risk. Twenty minutes a day of meaningful exercise, such as brisk walking, goes a long way to improving general health and reducing the risk of heart disease, stroke, and cancer.

The increase in body fat of much of the population has also been a cause of the cancer epidemic. Overweight people are at a significant increased risk for cancers and heart disease. The reason for the increased risk is not fully understood. The risk could be related to the type of food eaten, the lack of exercise, and perhaps most importantly to a general increase in inflammation of the body.

This type of inflammation is more complex than the inflammation that causes redness or swelling at sites of injury. Inflammatory molecules can effect a change in genes and gene function, as well as modify cell proteins. Perhaps the way that exercise, weight control, a good diet, and aspirin exert their benefit is through cooling down inflammation.

In the end, public health measures will likely finally end the cancer epidemic. In this regard, cancer medicine is about a decade behind advances in cerebrovascular medicine. The public health measures taken to reduce cerebrovascular disease, including blood pressure and cholesterol control, have been effective in decreasing the risk for developing heart and blood vessel disease. Disease specific treatment, including catheter-based procedures and surgical procedures, have become safer and more effective. The key observation of the role of abnormal blood clot formation called thrombosis, which blocks blood flow to the heart, brain, and other organs, led to the development of clot-preventing drugs and clot-destroying drug to treat the emergency complications of cerebrovascular disease and has improved outcomes.

I believe that equally effective measures will reduce the risk of developing cancer as the risk of heart disease and stroke have decreased. Further, those cancers not preventable by public health measures will be prevented and treated safely and effectively based on advances in cancer genetics and cancer care at the individual level. For now, though, we still must deal with cancer and its risks to health.

The diagnosis and treatment of cancer is complex. As illustrated, there are critical areas of cancer care where delays or mistakes can occur. Many patients do not have the financial means, even if they are fortunate enough to have insurance, to deal with the costs associated with cancer care.

It can often be difficult to obtain the best treatment for the patient, especially if the treatment is new or experimental. Insurance carriers can delay and deny medication and treatment authority, and can take the position that the treatment is not covered by the insurance contract. Such was the case of the young boy that I treated years ago for a recurrent leukemia. His initial treatment was given at a university hematology unit. Two years later the cancer recurred. His family could not travel to the university and I was asked by the family to take care of the child.

The leukemia was put into remission with additional chemotherapy. However, the child faced a high risk of yet another recurrence. I advised a bone marrow transplant using blood stem cells from a donor to take advantage of the vaccine-like effect of such an allotransplant. The transplant would be proceeded by high-dose chemotherapy. At the time, there was no bone marrow transplant in our state. The boy had relatives in another state and I located a transplant unit near their home so that he would have family to care for him during his treatment and recovery. He would need to stay for 100 days if all went well.

We were ready to proceed until I got a telephone call from the representative of the state medical office. The child's family had Medicaid coverage only and I was told that Medicaid would not cover the cost of the transplant because the office thought the procedure for this patient was experimental and too expensive and was to take place in another state. I was advised not to push the issue. I rejected the advise: I pushed it through and eventually approval came for the procedure. The young patient did very well with the treatment and his recovery.

Patients often receive their cancer diagnoses in an emergency room where they go for pain or other symptoms that may be chronic. This may complicate good cancer care. Too many times, cancers found during an emergency room visit are very far advanced and the patient is often already in poor health. Finding a cancer specialist with access to effective technologies can be difficult in that setting. For someone of limited means, finding an oncologist after discharge is challenging at best.

Despite the problems in the health care system today, the outlook for cancer prevention and treatment is positive. There are fewer people dying from cancer today than before because of better individualized treatments for those who do develop cancer. I can foresee a time when cancer prevention, diagnosis, and treatment will be readily accessible to all independent of the political aspects of our health care system. Cancer care will be inexpensive, effective and safe because of scientific advances in public health and medical care. Perhaps the future will include the techniques used by the fictional doctor "Bones" McCoy of the Star Trek series in diagnosing and treating patients. Using a handheld scanner the diagnosis will be made immediately and automated systems will treat the patient. Such a scanner may abrogate the need for an empathetic, skilled physician but until then, the doctor must serve the patient and family in multiple roles.

We will soon see most people living long, healthy, and active lives. With control of diseases such as cancer who knows how long a human life span can be. Until that time, the cancer journey has improved. The best outcomes will occur when the cancer patient, the family, and the cancer doctor find a human connection to one another that minimizes the anxiety and fear, and allows the patient to proceed confidently to the best diagnosis, treatment, and follow-up care.

My experience suggests that the initial first steps in effective cancer care and management is to find a knowledgeable, kind, and determined physician with access to good cancer care teams and modern technology. It might take several interviews to find such a person. There are many resources that can be used to find such care, including other family members, friends, or your place of worship. Ratings of cancer care providers are found on internet service sites and at the websites of the American Society of Clinical Oncologists (ASCO) and the American Society of Hematology (ASH). The oncologist you choose should be well schooled in the medical problems at hand, of course, but should also accept the responsibility of coordinating your care, fighting for you to get the best care possible and committed to providing ongoing care after the period of active treatment is completed. In short, your doctor should guide you through your entire cancer journey.

These stories illustrate the importance of freeing ourselves of the fear of cancer and promptly seeking help at the earliest stage. Cancer is, for patients and their families, a part of the challenge of life, a part of their human condition. This enemy can be successfully met and defeated.

Improvements in prevention, treatment and survivorship care are dramatic and available. Until the longed for end of cancer is here, we should be comforted by the reality that modern cancer medicine can cure many cancers and can provide real benefits for those suffering from cancers that cannot yet be cured. Cancer patients and their families deserve nothing less.